BROKEN TEMPLE

Rosemary Argente

During the Exodus on Mount Sinai

the Israelite built a movable temple

symbolic to the human body on its temporal sojourn

First edition 2018

Editor: Chris Wallace

Cover: Barry McDonald

Publishers: Asaina Books
Website: asainabooks.co.uk
Email: rosa@asainabooks.co.uk

Books by the same author:

Blantyre and Yawo Women
The Veil
The Promised Land - Companion to The Veil
Broken Temple
Praying Mantis
Difference
Share the Ride
Home From Home
Essays and Poetry
The Place Beyond
Caesar and Mapanga Homestead

Novels:
All Mine to Have
Farewell Sophomore
The Stream of Memory
A British Throne Scandal

Science Fiction:
Farewell to the Aeroplane

Booklets:
Journey of Discovery
Enduring Fountain - Health and Well-being
Katherine of the Wheel
Cooking With Asaina

For NHS Personnel

ACKNOWLEDGEMENTS

My sincere thanks are due to NHS personnel, those mentioned and those not mentioned in this book, for their kind and helpful answers to my questions during the preparation of the manuscript, and my thanks to Chris Wallace for editing the manuscript. My thanks are also due to Brian Sherman and Mark Sherman for their overall help in my struggles with computer technology.

CONTENTS

ONE

ON THE MORNING OF 25 JUNE 2015 – when I woke up – I felt totally alienated: I was 'here' yet I was not 'with it'. Friends, Yvonne and Clem, a couple I had not seen for a long time since my Bolton days, came along with Lorna, my daughter. I prepared a light lunch (as we were going out to Lorna and Archie's for dinner). We sat throughout the afternoon conversing as people do when they have not seen each other for a while, but the feeling of 'alienation' was getting more intense as the day wore on. Lorna collected us and we had a lovely dinner at their home as always (Lorna is a superb cook). Lorna took me home at 9 pm alone as the guests were staying with Lorna and Archie. She had offered to host them as she felt that I could not cope with looking after them – Lorna is always most considerate.

I immediately went to bed, I was tired. I woke up about an hour later as everything broke loose. I had no control over my waste matter. After clearing and clearing up I went back to bed. I woke up at 3:00 am, unable to shift the left side of my body. My left leg felt as if it was a piece of 'rubber' attached to me. I pressed the care line call button and mentioned that I believed I had a stroke. To my surprise Lorna came on line, but as I said everything was hazy; I had moved into the premises just five weeks before and was not familiar with the care call system. I said:

"I am sorry to call you at this hour. I think I have just had a stroke."

"I will call the Ambulance." She replied.

Promptly two ambulance men came along. The first thing they did was to test my blood pressure;

"Your blood pressure is very, very high!" Said one of the men.

"I do not suffer from high blood pressure", I protested.

"It is very high", he went on.

"It must be you handsome men raising my blood pressure!"

I hoped that I still had a sense of humour but if they thought they were confronting a 'nut case' I would not have blamed them. My mind and body were 'not at par' with my surroundings – there was no synchronisation. Past experience had taught me to succumb into the capable hands of 'medics'. I did not realise then that this was a farewell to the 'me' I had known till then, for my life was to change irreversibly, mentally and physically – I had a 'broken body'...

****

I WAS A LITTLE HAZY as to where the Ambulance took me, to the A & E or to Ward 7 of the Emergency Department. This is where one is assessed to determine where the patient should be sent to. Both are at the Dumfries & Galloway Royal Infirmary (DGRI) where they carried out various tests comprising blood pressure and blood sample - blood is perhaps the most important test (though other tests such as urine samples, temperature, oxygen levels, and others which they carried out are equally important), for blood is the currency of the Spiritual Realm (see *The Veil*, chapter 6, Science And Currency of the Spiritual Realm). [Note 1.]

At A & E or Ward 7, I was met by an amiable young doctor of Asian descent. After a few minutes he inquired about my ancestry, while the tests were being carried out. When I told him that one of the three parts of my ancestry was from my great, great grandfather who emigrated from Jamnagar (which borders Kashmir), India, to Africa, the Doctor went on:

"The people from that area are good-looking".

I could not imagine that after a stroke and the way I was feeling 'good-looking' could be applied to me! It must have been the Asian part of my descent that moved his question or he was just being kind since he was of an amiable disposition, not unlike most of the personnel there.

Note 1: A blood test is a quick and simple way to measure the amount of certain proteins, minerals, fats and sugars in one's blood. By looking at the levels of these in the blood, the doctor can find out how well the body is working and whether or not one has certain conditions or health problems. If first diagnosed with high blood pressure, the doctor or nurse may carry out one or more blood tests to help them plan the best treatment. This will show them as to whether there are certain factors present: if there is a raised cholesterol level; another medical problem, such as a kidney condition or diabetes; whether or not there is a problem with adrenal glands or kidneys and decide which medicines might work best for the patient. Body temperature is one of the four main vital signs that must be monitored to ensure safe and effective care. Temperature measurement is recommended by the National Institute of Clinical Excellence a part of the initial assessment in acute illness in adults (NICE, 2007) and by the Scottish Intercollegiate Guidelines Network guidelines for post-operative management in adults (SIGN, 2004). Despite applying in all healthcare environments, wide variations exist on the methods and techniques used to measure body temperature.

The conversation was going on while the various tests were being carried out: oximetry levels, oxygen levels through the process of pulse oximetry. This is very important because oxygen is vital to life and reduced levels of oxygen circulating in the bloodstream can lead to very serious, even fatal, complications for the heart, lung, brain and other organs. People with severe lung or heart disease, who are unconscious or who have difficulty breathing, or who need oxygen treatment for any reason are at risk of reduced oxygen levels, and consequently are at risk of serious illness. Urine sample (urinalysis) is a set of screening tests that can detect some common diseases. It may be used to screen for and/or help diagnose conditions such as a urinary tract infections, kidney disorders, liver problems, diabetes or other metabolic conditions, to name a few. Appropriate tests for all these were carried out.

The DGRI Emergency Department is open 24 hours (365 days a year). The Scottish Ambulance Service and Accident and Emergency departments provide care for people with symptoms of serious illness or who have been badly injured. When you call 999 the Scottish Ambulance Service will respond with the most appropriate help for your situation. Of all the NHS services, 999 and A&E are services that should only be used for serious illnesses or injuries. This means that essential treatment can be given to those who need it as quickly as possible.

The A & E is located in the DGRI, set in beautiful ever-green grounds (as most of Scotland) the District General Hospital serves the region of Dumfries and Galloway. The DGRI contains 337 staffed beds and has a full range of specialties.

****

THREE DAYS AFTER MY admission at DGRI my left eye felt as if something had got into it. I mentioned this to the Nurse who said that I would later be seen by an ophthalmologist. By the time they completed the tests it was the 27th and I was transferred to Ward 14 where there were many nurses, smiling, attentive and caring. I can best describe the experience in a poem in which I expressed my feelings:

Angels of Ward 14

They say angels dwell in heaven,
But where is Heaven?
Broken Body refuses to serve,
The paramedic says your blood pressure
is sky-high!
I don't suffer blood pressure high!
Paramedics raised my blood pressure sky-high!

At the emergency are many to welcome,
In the activity of medics in occupational vocation,
Each different, unique.
Mirrors of the soul, in varying eye colours,
Echoing some Hollywood great of yesteryear vocation,
But these are no mere actors.

Despite the absurdities of Broken Body,
All are ever patient, I thought I was the patient,
The beauty of our language spared.
All focused on the same goal:
Scans, X-rays, tests done, nothing spared,
To repair Broken Body.

Five star the sustenance scene,
Service with a smile, nothing too much trouble.
But we digress, who are the angels?
Where then is Heaven?
The caring compassionate scene,
There the angels are.

On the sixth day after the stroke I was discharged from Ward 14. Before being discharged I was told a number of things: I was not to drive for one month – what a punishment, not that I could drive anyway! That I should see an optician, and I was told that a Stroke Liaison Nurse would be assigned to me, and that she would make home visits after I left the hospital.

Lorna picked me up and took me home. I lived alone in a place where help would come at the press of a button - my daughter Lorna and her partner Archie lived five minutes away from me; and, I reminded myself that had my condition been that serious, they would most probably have assigned someone to look after me at home. Despite these assurances, I cannot pretend that I did not suffer some inexplicable 'fear'.

I was in "No Man's Land".

****

Monday 06 July 2015 -

ON THIS DAY Lorna, my daughter, took me to the ECG department at DGRI to attend my appointment for a Cardiac Ultrasound. This consisted of a cardiac examination. The heart is the vital part or essence in a human body, the driving engine if you like, which covers two aspects, the tangible and the intangible.

The tangible is the heart itself, a hollow muscular organ of vertebrate of the human body (and of animals) that by its rhythmic (without rhythm there is no life) contraction acts as a force pump maintaining the circulation of the blood. Like a dual acting engine, diastole and systole (contraction).

Diastole is the part of the cardiac cycle when the heart refills with blood following systole. Ventricular diastole is the period during which the ventricles are filling and relaxing, while atrial diastole is the period during which the atria are relaxing.

The intangible or intrinsic aspect of the heart involves feeling or feelings as in "heart of the matter", the core aspect of anything or condition in describing the quality aspect of something. Example: "the song touched the diastole and systole of my heart".

The most common heart ultrasound is non-invasive and very easy on the patient. A specially trained sonographer, uses a gel to slide a microphone-like device called a transducer over Stroke Liaison the chest area which allows reflected sound waves to provide a live picture of your heart and valves from the images. These measurements were to allow my Consultant and General Practitioner (GP) to make an informed decision on my future treatment.

****

I RECEIVED A LETTER by first class mail saying that an appointment had been arranged for me to attend the Community Rehabilitation at Nithbank (Rehab Nithbank). This is the place where treatment of disease, injury, or disability was dispensed by therapeutic interventions such as physiotherapy, occupational therapy, and nursing care rather than by drugs or surgery.

The goal of a stroke rehabilitation program is to help you relearn skills you lost when a stroke affected part of your brain. Stroke rehabilitation can help you regain independence and improve your quality of life. The programme can also help your brain get the job done. It may not reverse the effects of your stroke, but it can go a long way toward helping you regain your confidence and let you enjoy the things you love.

My appointment was arranged for 10:00 am at the Rehab Nithbank where I would be seen by the Community Rehabilitation Team. The appointment letter was in the regular format of the Dumfries and Galloway NHS Board which gave a telephone number (this format followed all other letters advising an appointment, among other communication details) to ring if one was unable to attend.

The letter also indicated that unless I contacted them to the contrary, the Patient Transport Service would collect me between 9 am and 10 am and would return me home at approximately 12 noon. It was signed by the Secretary of the Community Rehabilitation. I was still in "No Man's Land" and all that went with it when my 'Diary' commenced...

TWO

Wednesday 12 August 2015

I woke up with that feeling of 'expectancy', temporarily easing the fallacious phobia that had gripped me since I left the sanctuary of the hospital. My door bell rung at 9:30 am. (the bell is particularly loud and makes one jump! I have since placed a 'Welcome' note asking my visitors to knock instead). When I opened the door there were two Ambulance paramedics, a man and a pretty woman in their green uniform. Leaning on the man's strong arm and the pretty woman alongside, they escorted me to the Ambulance. Then up the hill we went, winding through a maze of bungalow-type buildings about four minutes drive from Nithsdale Mills, where I lived. The Ambulance stopped at the front entrance of the Rehab building. I noticed, when facing the entrance, on the right side were two high wooden boxes of flower blooms – a landmark as it were (I usually look for landmarks to aid my way to a new place).

We entered the double doors where immediately facing the entrance was the gateway to the Unit; a Reception window manned by Trevor Boulton (as I later learned his name). The ambulance medics led me to the left of the Reception through a door into the lounge area. I was received by a pretty, amiable hostess/nurse - these were my first impressions - and she bade me sit at a round table where other patients were seated. The area was surrounded by much information leaflets and other literature – including some used books for sale. As I was introduced to the other patients, I realised how fortunate I had been; for they appeared far more afflicted than I was.

I recalled what the consultant had said to me at Ward 14: "You had a wee stroke." The consultant had truly described my condition but in Scotland, even one's long signature becomes a "wee one" (a courtesy when making a request). The English equivalent of the seemingly 'understatement' can be distinguished from the Scottish one:

"He is not a bad player" when the footballer had just scored three goals! These are cultural differences found in all societies.

****

THE LEAD PLAYERS in their particular fields of expertise were: Gillian Young, Staff Nurse; and the Team: Senior Physiotherapist, Occupational Assistant; Occupational Therapist; Physiotherapy Assistant. All these medical *fundi* ('expert' in Swahili) help patients to develop, recover, and improve the skills needed for daily living and working.

We sat at the round table being entertained by the "hostess with the mostest" Christine Maxwell. Before the end of this session I discovered that she typically performed support activities, and she, in fact, was the Health Care Support Worker. She brought out some humour cards in between cups of tea, coffee and biscuits, as we awaited to be taken by a *fundi* in her particular field. The general atmosphere of the place was non-officious, friendly, like some kind of a 'social club', yet efficient. This was the place that carried out the process of repairing 'broken' Body (according to the Bible, Body is symbolised by a tabernacle or temple built by the Israelite on Sinai Desert during the Exodus, housing the soul on its temporal sojourn - see *The Veil,* chapter 7, Ministry of Yeshua, Body).

On this first day of my visit to the Rehab I was assessed by each of the Team and finally by Gillian who performed the *finale* interview of that morning's session.

From this day forward my inexplicable fear was dispelled. I had come from "No Man's Land" to the 'Safety Net' of the Dumfries Community Rehabilitation at Nithbank.

****

AFTER OBSERVING THE HIGH standards achieved by the modern medical world, my thoughts took me to my childhood when I was three and went to live with my grandmother Asaina, at her Yawo village where she was the Matriarch ('Anganga', grandmother in the Yawo language. [Note 2.]

Note 2: The Anganga was trained by her grandmother to be a qualified herbalist healer, a qualification that was always attached to the position of 'Matriarch' and passed down over the generations from mother to daughter (matrilineal society). She was familiar with the traditional healing methods comprised of roots or bark of certain trees (soaked in water); and leaves of certain trees and other foliage. These healed most ailments, particularly those suffered by children: such as fever, malaria, colds, sore throats, mumps and others: including serious conditions such as epilepsy, asthma, black water fever, and cancerous sores. A medical service that knew no surgery, consequently a good number of mothers died in childbirth for lack of the knowledge of caesarian section birth. (See booklet *Enduring Fountain – Health and Well-being*).

Worthy of note is that an individual survives in any community or society by its current mode of services, whatever those services may be, which endure up to the time of the individual's demise. At this stage I had never seen a Western European doctor. I was five when I came across one at the Church of Scotland Mission Hospital, Blantyre, Malawi, after I had joined my parents and brother. And, during my early teens Dr Dabb, the first ever female doctor in the country, was assigned to the Blantyre Mission Hospital. She was Scottish.

ABOUT TWO WEEKS after I was discharged from Ward 14, I experienced similar symptoms to those on the day I had the stroke. An Ambulance was called. The Ambulance medic checked my blood pressure and said because he had detected some connection with a 'heart' condition, I was to be taken to the hospital. But then, again on this occasion everything was 'hazy'.

I was taken to Ward 7 where they carried out tests when I was told that I had a TIA [Note 3], which sometimes occurred and often lasted for less than five minutes caused by a temporary decrease in blood supply to the brain. I was sent home after 24 hours.

Note 3: It may be helpful to try and understand what a stroke is. A stroke occurs when the blood supply to one's brain is interrupted or reduced. A stroke is a brain attack similar to a heart attack, and is mostly caused by a blockage of a blood vessel to part of the brain. In a minority of cases it can be caused by an area of bleeding into the brain, referred to as an haemorrhagic stroke and should be treated as a medical emergency. This deprives the brain of oxygen and nutrients, which can cause the brain cells to die. A stroke may be caused by a blocked artery (ischemic stroke) or the leaking or bursting of a blood vessel (haemorrhagic stroke). Some people may experience only a temporary disruption of blood flow to their brain (transient ischemic attack, or TIA). About 85 percent of strokes are ischaemic strokes (IS) which occur when the arteries to one's brain become narrower or blocked, causing severely reduced blood flow (ischaemia). When this happens, the brain does not get enough oxygen or nutrients which causes brain cells to die. Strokes occur due to problems with the blood supply to the brain; either the blood supply is blocked or a blood vessel within the brain raptures. There are three main kinds of stroke, ischaemic, haemorrhagic and TIA. [See Addendum.]

I WAS SOON VISITED at my home by Karen Smith who was allocated to me as the "Home Visiting Stroke Nurse". She assisted me in more ways than one. She was most helpful on checking various aspects connected with my progress to better health. Karen gave me much advise including information on the services of Age Concern. She also recommended that I see an optician at Boots, as they would be in a position to tell me as to when I would be able to drive again.

As I have said before, the NHS care covered the whole body from head to toe. A dentist had been recommended by Gillian who gave me a card for Great King Street Dental, located in a street of the same name. When the month of 'forbidden to drive' had been over, I first decided to attend to the issue of seeing an optician and since I was not allowed to drive, I got a taxi and went to Boots opticians. My eyes were tested, my glasses updated, and I was given the 'all clear' to drive verdict. It was so good to be back behind the wheel.

****

SOON AFTER MY ADMISSION at the Rehab Nithbank I was able to move about and Lorna took me to the Dumfries & Galloway Multi Cultural Centre in Hollywood House, Irish Street. Among other people I met there was Venus Alae-Carew, an active member of the Bahá'í community. Bahá'í Faith is a world religion whose purpose is to unite all the races and peoples in one universal Cause and whose members strive for continuing personal, professional and spiritual development, and for effective service to humanity. There are no priests or pastors in the Bahá'í Faith. So in the Bahá'í community everyone is a member in the 'humble posture of learning' and 'striving day by day that their actions may become beautiful prayers' [Note 4.]

One of the most interesting persons I met at the gatherings of

Venus was Ann-Marie Budyn, JP (Justice of the Peace). She struck me as a rather 'worldly' person. [We shall meet her again in chapter 6).

Note 4:   As no one has a position as such as there is no hierarchy. However, those who have had the bounty and time to train, would become tutors in the curriculum designed specifically to raise capacity for spiritual development and service to the community, so in that sense Venus is a tutor for the Training Institute trying to learn about creating vibrant local communities. Also when there are a larger number of registered Baha'i members, the communities are engaged to forming Administrative bodies and locally they are   called 'Local Spiritual Assembly', and they are formed by local elections. Continued below...

August 2015 – Rehab Nithbank
It had been decided that my weekly attendance at the Rehab Nithbank was to be set for Wednesdays. I was collected by the same Ambulance with the man and lovely young woman and taken to the Rehab Nithbank. On this occasion each of the *fundi* carried out the essential exercises proper. The Senior Physiotherapist, performed and showed me the exercises I was to do at home consisting of physical exercises mostly on my legs.

The Occupational Assistant, was directly involved in providing therapy, mainly to my hands. The Occupational Therapist, was also involved in my hands using a yellow-coloured putty to kneed with my left hand (the stroke had weakened the left side of my body). She aided and typically performed support. The Physiotherapy Assistant (PTA) was a health care worker who helped me effectively to cope with my limitations in movement, daily functioning and activity. She worked under the supervision of the physiotherapist.

****

Wednesday 26 August 2015 – Rehab Nithbank

I was again collected by the Ambulance, though I was back to driving they never asked me to drive there myself. The therapy on my legs and hands continued. The plan for this day was initially to see me in CRU for activities to assess hand strength and function. The activities were carried out in the treatment room to assess fine finger movement. I managed well with transferring small pegs across on to the peg board with a good range of movement. The benefits of retrograde massage was explained and carried out on my left hand with cream. Also carried out was activity with yellow putty, rolling out with fingers and increased opposition with fingers. I was given putty and ball to practice at home. I also practised with large coloured pegs with each finger and

****

Note 4 continued: The Bahá'í Faith was founded by Bahá'u'lláh in the mid-nineteenth century in Persia, from where he was exiled for his teachings to the Ottoman Empire. He died while officially still a prisoner at Akka. The Bahá'í Faith in Scotland is a minority religion. According to the 2001census in Scotland, about four hundred people living in Scotland declared themselves to be Bahá'ís, compared to a 2004 figure of approximately 5,000 Bahá'ís in the United Kingdom. Scotland's Bahá'í history began around 1905 when European visitors, Scots among them, (including Continued below:

thumb which I managed well but there was some weakness with my hand in handling the black pegs.

I soon received a home visit to assess a toilet transfer with 2" raised toilet seat and assess the use of a kitchen trolley.

****

ON THE REVERSE SIDE of most appointment letters called for a list of medication one had been prescribed: I had been prescribed Clopidogrel, Atorvastatin, and Amlodipine, while I was in Ward 14 right at the outset and I was to take them for the rest of my life. Clopidogrel is a blood-thinning medication that helps to prevent clots forming in your blood and to reduce the risk of heart disease and stroke in those at high risk; often prescribed after a transient ischaemic attack (TIA) or an ischaemic stroke to help reduce one's risk of having another ischaemic stroke or TIA. Atorvastatin is a member of the drug category known as 'statins', which are used primarily as a lipid-lowering agent and for prevention of events associated with cardiovascular disease. Amlodipine is a calcium channel blocker that dilates (widens) blood vessels and improves blood flow and is used to treat chest pain (angina) and other conditions caused by coronary artery disease. Amlodipine is also used to treat high blood pressure(hypertension). For the first three months of taking these medications my bed linen was covered in blood. [Note 5]

****

Note 4 continued: Mrs Jane Elizabeth Whyte of Charlotte Square, Edinburgh) met 'Abdu'l-Bahá, the eldest son of Bahá'u'lláh and then the head of the religion, in Ottoman Palestine. One of the first and most prominent Scots who became a Baha'i was Dr John Esslemont from Aberdeen. In the 1920's he wrote Baha'u'llah And the New Era: An Introduction to the Baha'i Faith which is still in print and widely read. The Bahá'í communities are well known for their inter-faith activities in Scotland.
"It is not for him to pride himself who loveth his own country, but rather for him who loveth the whole world. The earth is but one country, and mankind its citizens." Bahá'u'lláh' *Gleanings from the Writings of Baha'u'llah*, p. 94.
Note 5: My blood type is Rh D Negative. In my research I discovered that there are only 9.7% of this type out of 7.6 billion people on Planet Earth (census of 2018, see *The Place Beyond*, Epilogue, and *The Veil*, chapter 6, Genealogy of Yeshua, Conception, Science, and Currency of the Spiritual Realm). While my blood type caused the loss of my infants in the early

1950s, it also saved my life when I was deliberately poisoned in 1985.

Wednesday 02 September 2015 – Rehab Nithbank
I attended CRU [please spell out CRT, CRU, and OTA] and joint intervention of Tai Chi in sitting position was carried out. I was able to follow instructions consistently though I was fatigued before the end. Before I attended on the above date I was called to the Rehab, Nithbank for a one day assessment to see how I was getting on.

At every one of these sessions the usual 'social club' general atmosphere of the place prevailed, in between waiting for therapy appointments/ interviews, at the 'round table'. This made the visits to the Rehab an enjoyable social outing.

****

Tuesday 26 October 2015 – Gym at the Crichton
IT WAS ARRANGED FOR ME to attend the Stroke Exercises at the Rehabilitation, Crichton Royal Hospital where I met the Lead Physiotherapist in Stroke Rehabilitation and her Team. My first appointment was at 1:00 pm, set on Tuesdays. By this time I was back behind the wheel and did not need anyone to take me or for me to order a taxi.

Some of the exercises conducted were similar to what I had when I lived in Bolton (see *Home From Home*) where I faithfully attended for four years and continued to do them at home at least four times a week, which involved, standing, and sitting. To these I added exercises shown to me by a physiotherapist when I had been involved in a car accident, which entailed exercising on the floor. [Note 6.]

When I inquired about floor exercises at the Gym, I was told:
   "We never ask people to go on the floor."

Note 6: The spinal cord is protected by the vertebral column, also known as the spinal column or backbone. The human spinal column is made up of 33 bones. 7 vertebrae in the cervical region, 12 in the thoracic region, 5 in the lumbar region, 5 in the sacral region and 4 in the coccyx region. I was involved in a car accident (whiplash 1992) and my lower back was injured. The pain in my spine increased after the stroke and I was unable to park my Nissan automatic car in everse. It was easier and less painful to reverse out of a parking space as I could use the mirrors to see where I was going (it was fitted with an audio warning if one got too close to some object). After the whiplash, a Chiropractor had taken X-rays of my back and discovered that I had one extra bone in my spinal column and this prevented me from bending backward.

I have always been a great believer in the value of exercising and I commenced exercising when I was fifteen. From that age I wanted to become an Acrobat, just for my own pleasure not to entertain as in the circus! For some unknown reason I could not bend backwards. I could go forward, while lying down and bring my toes over my head to touch the floor. I was envious of the children who could bend back and touch the floor without any trouble at all.

While I was attending the programmes on Wednesdays at the Rehab Nithbank and the stroke class on Tuesdays, the outpatients appointments in between were endless covering my entire body from head to toe, they missed out nothing!

Wednesday 11 November 2015 – Rehab Nithbank - Recall
I RECEIVED THE USUAL LETTER telling me of my recall appointment (on above date) indicating that this would give the Team a chance to see how I had been coping since my last attendance; and to review any changes in my therapy needs. At this meeting I answered the Team's questions on my recreation, mainly driving; that I had no falls; and that I was managing my ADLs (activities of daily living such as daily self care "the things we normally do such as feeding ourselves, bathing, dressing,
grooming, work, homemaking, and leisure"). I explained that

my main difficulty was chopping vegetables due to increasing arthritic pain in my hands, but that I had found a solution by buying pre-prepared vegetables. They also inquired about my upcoming Orthopaedic appointment (as indicated in previous chapters they had a finger on all my health needs!). I also indicated that I had obtained a private cleaner to assist with household tasks. The plan was to await the Orthopedic review and recall in January 2016 at the Rehab Nithbank.

****

Saturday 14 November 2015 – Audiology

AS INDICATED PREVIOUSLY that they 'left nothing' out but ensured that every aspect of the human body was functioning properly, and my next 'in between' appointment was for the above. Audiology is the branch of science and medicine concerned with the sense of hearing, balance and related disorders. For many years prior to the above date I had been using hearing aids prescribed because of tinnitus (ringing or buzzing in the ears, a subjective matter within one's head and not an external factor) which had been bothering me for some time. In Audiology I attended the DGRI in Bankend Road and it was a matter of updating my existing hearing aids.

****

Ophthalmology
Monday 14 December 2015

I INDICATED IN CHAPTER 1 that three days after my stroke while I was at the DGRI, I felt a "little something" in my left eye. This little something remained throughout the days that followed. It was not painful but just a little irritating factor. Though when I placed my hand on my right eye I could not read anything with my left eye (for many years I have needed glasses only for reading, as my distant sight was always good enough to see the horizon).

From the above mentioned date of appointment there were further nine appointments where the tests were carried out by different members of the Ophthalmology team (I have explained in my Postscript E the nature and importance of "team work").

From the above mentioned date of appointment there were further nine appointments when the tests were carried out by different members of the Ophthalmology team (I have explained in my Postscript E the nature and importance of "team work"). These entailed eye drops and photos taken of my eyes. The finding was that the eyesight was already going weak and the stroke merely accelerated it. Also, my GP was requested to prescribe Systane eye drops which I was to apply three times a day. At a later appointment, after carrying out more tests and photos taken, it was said of my left eye that it could possibly end up worse off after surgery, and that an option was a cataract surgery (a medical condition in which the lens of the eye becomes progressively opaque, resulting in blurred vision).

****

I SOON VISISTED THE HOME   of Venus at her invitation where she held regular meetings (alternatively hosted by other Bahá'í members in their homes). My meeting with her was to enrich and expand my social and spiritual life, for through her I met many interesting people from different walks of life. What I personally found interesting and desirable in the Bahá'í Faith was their belief in the indestructible values: love, peace, unity, justice, and charity which closely follow the teachings of Jesus. [Note 7.]

One of the most interesting persons I met at the gatherings of Venus was Ann-Marie Budyn. She was a JP (Justice of the Peace) and she struck me as rather 'worldly'. (We shall meet her again in chapter 5.)

****

Tuesday 04 July 2017 at 8:15

I received the usual appointment letter telling me that an Admission to Hospital – Day Care (Ward 17) was arranged for the above date. Along with this was an information sheet on the usual things on pre "Do and Don't". Post operative refraction record.

Then I met the Consultant (*fundi*) who was to carry out the surgery. The gentlest of hands prepared me for the surgery before the Consultant was to commence his task; and a nurse sat next to me holding my hands and told me that I should squeeze her hand should I feel any pain.

Another nurse was on my right, and I believe the *fundi* was behind my head. I thought I was still waiting for the surgery to be carried out; for I felt no pain or discomfort whatsoever. Then it was over.

Another letter followed this telling me that I was to attend the hospital the following day (Wednesday 05 July). On this day a "reading test" was carried out on my left eye to start with. It was not a matter of: "I see", said the blind man (as he hit a lamp post!) but it was like a "window opened to the world". I could read the Eye Chart. A miracle had been performed!

Note 7: Jesus was the Word. He was as the station of reality compared to the station of metaphor. There is no intrinsic meaning in the leaves of a book, but the thought they convey leads you to reflect upon reality. The reality of Jesus was the perfect meaning, the Christhood in Him which in the Holy Books is symbolized as the Word.

When asked on one occasion: 'What is a Bahá'í?' Abdu'l-Bahá replied: "To be a Bahá'í simply means to love all the world; to love humanity and try to serve it; to work for universal peace and universal brotherhood."

THREE

MY MEDICAL HOME BASE is St Michael's Medical Centre, and my appreciation is also for the tremendous, courteous, and outstanding help extended to me by the personnel of St Michael's Medical Centre, more so after the stroke I had (25/06/15). In particular I highly commend the outstanding courtesy of my personal GP for his untiring and persistent efforts in making certain that every aspect of my medical needs was met and rectified.

What I noted particularly in all the NHS departments that cared for me, was that they all dispensed their services through "team work", which in another word is "Unity". [Note 8.]

The place where I took up residence since my move to Dumfries in 2015, was Nithsdale Mills, sheltered/retirement/supported housing for older people, very well run by Loreburn Housing Association. The Care Call service which they operate is reassuring.

****

Wednesday 02 September 2015 – Rehab Nithbank
I attended CRU [please spell out CRT, CRU, and OTA] and joint intervention of Tai Chi in sitting position was carried out. I was able to follow instructions consistently though I fatigued at the end.
Before I attended on the above date I was called to the Rehab, Nithbank for a one day assessment to see how I was getting on.
At every one of these sessions the usual 'social club' general atmosphere of the place prevailed, in between waiting for

therapy appointments/ interviews, at the 'round table'. This made the visits to the Rehab like some enjoyable social outing.

****

Note 8: The best way I can describe the NHS "team work" which in another word is 'Unity' is by quoting 'Abdu'l-Baha', eldest son and successor of Baha'u'llah, the founder of the Baha'i Faith:

"Those who are working alone are like ants, but when they are united they will become as eagles. Those who work singly are as drops, but, when united, they will become a vast river carrying the cleansing water of life into the barren desert places of the world. Before the power of its rushing flood, neither misery, nor sorrow, nor any grief will be able to stand... (Lady Blomfield, *The Chosen Highway*, p. 171)"

"So powerful is the light of unity it can illuminate the whole earth.." Baha'u'llah...(1817–1892).

Wednesday 09 September 2015 - Rehab Nithbank

ON THIS OCCASION I was told of the planned task of assessing fine finger movement (note: they always explained in advance what they were going to do and obtained one's consent there and then). My pain was at the base of my right hand below the thumb. I pointed out that the pain was similar to possible arthritic pain I had previously experienced with my left hand (which gave me a permanent crooked thumb. Since over twenty years ago following Margaret Hill's remedy for daily intake of cider vinegar, no more limbs have become crooked, see *Enduring Fountain – Health and Well-being*) and I had been unable to use at home the putty I had been given. On this occasion exercises were carried out on my left hand for fine finger movement using small pieces with a solitaire board. I managed well with grasping and using all fingers.

It was a repeat of the usual pleasantness and I took the occasion to mention that I was back 'behind the driving wheel' since my stroke (driving for me over the years gets

23

'the blues on the run' to the point of euphoria!). However, the difference on this occasion was that I missed Gillian as she was away. The usual person who stood in for her to perform the *finale* of the morning's session was the Manager of the Community Rehabilitation Unit/Continence Team. I met Chris Wallace, a person with a caring disposition and an unassuming countenance. The interview took place in the well-designed spacious kitchen of the Rehab Nithbank, adjacent to the lounge area. Chris offered me a drink but I had already had my cup of coffee at the round table amid the usual 'amusements'. His questions were more general on my progress towards better health, and the usual small talk people engaged in at an initial meeting.

Over the years, it has been natural for me to express my feelings through poetry on things that have deeply touched me. The expression of my feelings and understanding of the Rehabilitation at Nithbank lies in the following poem:

Angels of Rehab
They say angels dwell in heaven,
    But where is Heaven?
    Broken Body refuses to serve.
    The ambulance paramedics call for the Rehab,
    The man's strong arm to lean on
    The pretty girl along, both in green uniform.

At the Rehab are many to welcome,
    Each different, unique but in Grace uniform:
    By decorum in conduct,
    Refinement in acquiescence,
    Kind, self-less, caring,
    But this is no jargon of descent.

The caring compassionate place,

A social club seemingly, yesterday dominoes,
Today the humour cards to amuse,
In-between tea, coffee and biscuits.
I espy Frank Sinatra of yesteryear
The manager I am told.

Oops! I digressed to yesteryear,
  But who are the Angels? Where are they?
  At the caring compassionate place,
  All focused on the same thing,
  To repair Broken Body,
  There the Angels are...

****

Wednesday 16 September 2015 – Rehab Nithbank

As usual I was collected by the ambulance and at the Rehab Unit I was told that this therapy session was for finger movements. At this stage I was still having the arthritic pains in both hands, and I had not used the putty because of this. I pointed out that my left hand had become stronger than the right hand. I was told to continue with the putty at home provided there was no swelling.

****

Wednesday 23 September 2015

ON THIS OCCASION it was to review finger exercises. I advised the therapist that I had been using the thera putty once every day and doing finger exercises. At this session I rolled out putty using all fingers, and the session was good. There was grasp and strength in my left hand with the thera putty; continued activity with pegs; lifted all coloured pegs from board using all fingers and thumb and transferred pegs back onto board, though I was unable to transfer the black pegs.

This was followed by an appointment on the 30th September for an informal review by the Staff Nurse.

****

Thursday 30 September 2015
BY THIS TIME I was much behind the wheel though I was still collected by the ambulance. The letter giving the date of appointment (above date) indicated that there was to be an informal review meeting to discuss my progress, and also indicated that I could bring a member of my family if I so wished. The usual exercises, which preceded the interview, were more like a review of my progress. As usual the *finale* was carried out by Gillian, the Staff Nurse. She took my blood pressure and weight. I was told that they were pleased with my progress and I was to be discharged that morning to return in 4-6 weeks time.

For a good number of years whenever my blood pressure was taken, for some unknown reason, the pressure was always high. This may have been due to a combination of things, the main one being anxiety. I came to realise that on the third take the pressure registered 'normal' though this situation changed since I was prescribed Amlodipine, when my blood pressure was normal on the first take. This medication belongs to a group of medicines called calcium antagonists. It is used to treat: high blood pressure (hypertension), angina pectoris (pain in the chest caused by blockages in the arteries to the heart) or chest pain classed as vasospatic angina pectoris or Prinzmetal's angina.

****

Tuesday 26 October 2015 – Stroke Rehab Gym exercises
IT HAD BEEN ARRANGED FOR ME to attend the Stroke Rehabilitation Exercises at the Crichton Royal Hospital

(Rehab Crichton) where I met the Leader and her Team. My first appointment was at 1:00 pm, set on Tuesdays. By this time I was back behind the wheel and did not need anyone to take me or for me to order a taxi. This was followed by other dates of attendance.

I found the exercises at the Rehab Crichton to be most beneficial. Regular exercise ensures a healthy lifestyle; it can help one sleep better; and feel more energised during the day. Engaging in regular physical activity can do a number of things as studies show the benefits it can
have such as help one to manage one's weight and reduce the risk of developing certain diseases, help prevent mental health problems, including type 2 diabetes and high blood pressure. Exercise has favourable effects on the pain that is associated with various conditions, also increases pain tolerance, and your brain and body can do more. You are not winded walking upstairs, and your heart rate and blood pressure decrease.

The exercises were not unlike what I had before when I lived in Bolton where I joined Get Active (see *Home From Home*) where I faithfully attended exercise classes for four years. But then I have always been a great believer in the benefits of regular exercising. I commenced exercising when I was fifteen. The point being that from that age I wanted to become an Acrobat (just for my pleasure not to entertain as in the circus!) but for some inexplicable reason I could not bend backwards. I could only go forward, lie down and bring my toes over my head to touch the floor but never backward. I was envious of the children who could bend back and touch the floor without any trouble at all, particularly children of the village.

Many years later when I had back pains caused by whiplash

injury in a car accident (1996), a Chiropractor took X-rays of my back. It was discovered that I had one extra bone in my spinal column and this prevented me from bending backward (see *The Place Beyond*, Epilogue, and Note 5). At the time a physiotherapist showed me how to deal with the back pain by doing exercises that involved going on the floor. I have faithfully carried out these exercises which I combine with the exercises shown to me at the Rehab Nithbank and the Stroke Rehab, Crichton as my "home exercises".

However, it became necessary for me to have certain surgeries (as will be seen in appropriate dates and chapters of this text). After each surgery I felt very tired and was unable to do any exercises for at least three days, regardless of the fact that the surgeries were painless. Consequently, I found it difficult to use my body as it increasingly felt like it was a piece of 'heavy rock' I could not manage. It was during this time that I came fully to realise the importance of daily exercising.

However, equally important is 'resting'. That is to say one should alternate exercises with a time to rest. [Note 9.]

****

26 October 2015 - Dental appointment

IN CHAPTER 2 I indicated that the Staff Nurse gave me a card on a recommended dentist and I made an appointment on the above date to see the Great King Street Dentist in the street of the same name. This was one of my 'in between' appointments during my attendance at the Rehab Nithbank.

According to my observation, I found that all the NHS departments I was invited to attend to improve my health applied "team work". [see Note 8]

While I was attending the programmes on Wednesdays at the Rehab Nithbank and the stroke class on Tuesdays, the outpatients appointments in between were endless covering my entire body from head to toe, they missed out nothing!

****

Wednesday 11 November 2015 – Rehab Nithbank - Recall
I RECEIVED THE USUAL LETTER telling me of my recall appointment (on above date) indicating that this would give the Team a chance to see how I had been coping since my last attendance; and to review any changes in my therapy needs. At this meeting I answered the Team's questions on my recreation, mainly driving; that I had no falls; my ADLs (activities of daily living such as daily self care "the things we normally do such as feeding ourselves, bathing, dressing, grooming, work, homemaking, and leisure"). I explained that my main difficulty was chopping vegetables due to increasing arthritic pain in my hands, but

Note 9: Since I was age 45 I resolved to take a *siesta* every day which I found most helpful in renewed energy to get on with things. I copied this from Winston Churchill who, when he became Britain's Prime Minister for most of World War II (1940-1945), took a daily ten-minute nap after lunch in his chair, he was then refreshed to think out the war strategy - it was that nap that won the War! In life we all fight a kind of private war.

that I had found a solution by buying ready-prepared vegetables. They also inquired about my upcoming Orthopaedic appointment (as indicated in previous chapters they had a finger on all my health needs!). I also indicated that I had obtained a private cleaner to assist with household tasks. The plan was to await the Orthopaedic review and recall in January 2016 at the Rhab Nithbank.

29

Saturday 14 November 2015 – Audiology

AS INDICATED PREVIOUSLY that they 'left nothing' out but ensured that every aspect of the human body was functioning properly, and my next 'in between' appointment was for the above. Audiology is the branch of science and medicine concerned with the sense of hearing, balance and related disorders. For many years prior to the above date I had been using hearing aids prescribed because of tinnitus (ringing or buzzing in the ears, a subjective matter within one's head and not an external factor) which had been bothering me for some time. In Audiology I attended the DGRI in Bankend Road and it was a matter of updating my existing hearing aids.

****

27 November 2015 - Orthotics

AS I HAVE INDICATED IN PREVIOUS CHAPTERS there were in-between appointments on matters besides the Rehabilitation attendance. I received the usual letter of Appointment telling me that an appointment had been arranged for me on the above date at the Orthotics/Orthopaedic Department. The letter indicated that I was to be seen by one of the members of the Team. There I met other members of the Team. Both my feet were examined, my footprints were made on foam, and measurements were taken for a pair of shoes; and was told that later for ankle boots.

Like fingerprints, every single person's foot is unique. Over the counter premoulded/self forming orthotics are simply gimmicks that cause more discomfort than relief because they don't fit one's unique arch. Only footprint insole technology achieve true lab level customisation (I recall that I could not wait for my age of 18 to be allowed to wear high heels shoes! In high heels shoes one is literally walking with the forehead, according to reflexology).

****

Monday 14 December 2015 - Ophthalmology

I SAID IN CHAPTER ONE that three days after my stroke while I was at the DGRI, I felt a "little something" in my left eye. This little something remained throughout the days that followed. It was not painful but just an irritating little *gremlin.* Though when I placed my hand on my right eye my vision was blurred let alone read anything with my left eye (for many years I have needed glasses only for reading, as my distant sight had always been good enough to see the horizon).

From the above mentioned date of appointment there were further nine appointments where the tests were carried out by different members of the Ophthalmology team (I have explained in Postscript E the nature and importance of "team work"). These entailed eye drops and photos taken of my eyes.

The finding was that the eyesight in the left eye was already going weak before the stroke. Also, my GP was requested to prescribe Systane eye drops which I was to apply three times a day. At a later appointment, after carrying out more tests and photos taken, it was said of my left eye that it could possibly end up worse off after surgery, and that an option was cataract surgery (a medical condition in which the lens of the eye becomes progressively opaque, resulting in blurred vision) to be carried out in both eyes.

FOUR

Thursday 21 January 2016 – Occupational Therapy
OCCUPATIONAL THERAPY (OT) is the use of particular activities as an aid to recuperation from physical or mental illness. OT is a client-centred health profession concerned with promoting health and well being through occupation. The primary goal of occupational therapy is to enable people to participate in the activities of everyday life. Occupational therapists achieve this outcome by working with people and communities to enhance their ability to engage in the occupations they want to, need to, or are expected to do, or by modifying the occupation or the environment to better support their occupational engagement.

****

Wednesday 09 February 2016 – Rehab Nithbank, Recall
I RECEIVED THE USUAL LETTER that a recall/review appointment had been arranged for me on the above date to see how I had been coping since my last attendance and to review any changes in my therapy needs.

I was seen jointly by the Senior Physiotherapist, Occupational Assistant; Occupational Therapist; and Physiotherapy Assistant. I explained that I was managing well at home and regularly getting about in my car but that I had occasional pain in my joints and spine (see Note 7) which resulted in headaches; that my GP was aware of the situation and he prescribed pain relief; and that I still felt fatigued but managed this by my usual *siesta* (afternoon rest or nap see Postscript H). There were no concerns raised at this session and I was discharged from the Rehab Nithbank. A letter was sent to my GP explaining the situation.

****

07 April 2016 – Physiotherapy

I WAS GIVEN AN APPOINTMENT on the above date. Physiotherapy deals with the treatment of disease, injury, or deformity by physical methods such as massage, heat treatment, and exercise rather than by drugs or surgery. This included Pelvic Floor Exercises (the muscular-base of the abdomen, attached to the bony pelvis). These exercises are very important. They protect against symptoms of pelvic insufficiency, restore pelvic well being, improve intimate sensations, boost self-esteem and confidence, but above all they help to maintain 'continence' (Latin *continentia* meaning 'holding back').

I had always been conscious of a 'healthy lifestyle' particularly commencing in 1972 (eight years before I left Malawi for Britain) when I had a dietary problem caused by fresh cow's milk. On the advice of my GP, it was then I switched to soy milk (in those days only available in powder form). This strengthened my conviction to study food values and the result was my booklet *Enduring Fountain – Health and Well-being*, which commences with a poem and the sentences: *"We are: What we eat. What we drink. What we think. What we do."*

Monday 18 April 2016 - SpecSavers

I ATTENDED SPECSAVERS on a Recall/Review appointment for my glasses. I was told that I had to wait for the Consultant's decision on what was to be done to my left eye (and possibly to my right eye as well) before they could update my glasses. However, they prescribed a temporary pair of glasses but these were not of much use for reading as they were not 'balanced'. I felt as if my eyes were set at 'different' levels.

****

ON MAY 2016 I had purchased a Nissan Note automatic car which was delivered to me in Dumfries by Church Wharf Garage from Bolton, the garage that provided me with excellent motor services for 18 years (see *Home From Home*). This meant I did not need to hire a taxi, save the Rehab attendance when I was collected by ambulance. In my entire 68 years of driving, at this stage, this was the second ever automatic car I had, for in an automatic car I never felt that I was 'driving'. Nonetheless, my Nissan gave me the confidence I needed in driving expertise given my current condition – a stroke forever changes one's life, physically as mentally and this car had all the gadgets to suit a physically challenged person.

****

Friday 22 April 2016 – Radiology
I HAD SEEN MY GP on the pain at the back of my neck. Since I had rheumatic fever in 1986 I had been much bothered by osteoarthritis (I have never tried to discover if the two were in any way connected).
Radiology is the science dealing with X-rays and other high-energy radiation, especially the use of such radiation for the diagnosis and treatment of disease. A cervical spine X-ray is a safe and painless test that uses a small amount of radiation to take a picture of the bones in the back of the neck (cervical vertebrae).

This was followed up by by two other Radiology appointments on 09 June 2016 and 20 September to carry out an X-ray of the pelvis focused specifically on the area between one's hips that holds many of reproductive and digestive organs. This was requested by my GP due to the pain in my hip.

****

Wednesday 10 August 2016 – Orthotics
I RECEIVED THE USUAL LETTER advising me that an appointment had been arranged for the above date; and I was to be seen by the lead player or a member of her Team. I was also requested to take my footwear to the appointment for review. I left the shoes there as they were too tight and was given a date when to collect a corrected pair.

This appointment was followed by other two appointments on Tuesday 05 September and 20 September with the usual appointment letter that I would be seen by one of the members of the Team. I collected my shoes and this time they were perfect. On the second appointment I was examined for ankle boots. There followed other appointments in 2016, on 24th October, 14 November 2016; and then again on 14 December 2016.
At these appointments various things were done and questions asked but mostly to see how I fared with the shoes that had been issued to me.

For orthotics to work effectively it is essential that the shoes in which they are worn have the following features: Extra depth at the toes and the heel to allow the foot to fit comfortably into the shoe. Shoes with removable insoles have increased depth and so are preferred by podiatrists when fitting orthotics. In my case it was a matter of getting shoes that would improve my balance in walking.

****

Thursday 11 August 2016

I INDICATED IN CHAPTER ONE that I was soon visited by Karen Smith, Stroke Nurse who arranged for a good number of things. One of the things she organised was for me to receive most helpful literature from Age Scotland which carried the slogan: *Love Later Life,* a Scottish charity. The information came under several headings, each with a number of subheadings on useful information covering every aspect of one's existence, including legal and family issues. This included literature covering various aspects all designed to maintain a healthy lifestyle, particularly reducing the risk of stroke. The literature was comprised of Silver Letters, a wholly independent Scottish charity, *Stroke Series* SS3; *Chest, Heart and Stroke Scotland*; and Silver Line UK (founded by Dame Esther Rantzen).

****

Wednesday 23 November 2016

I VISITED MY GP and explained that I was having problems with swallowing. I was referred to the Adult Speech & Language Therapy where I was seen by a member of the Team and I was given several exercises and literature to enable me to carry out the exercises at home. The literature was comprehensive: listing appropriate foods to eat and foods to be avoided. Interestingly, this included the Mendelson Manoeuvre, which is a swallowing manoeuvre designed to treat both reduced laryngeal (speech sound) excursion and limited cricopharyngel (relating to the cricoid cartilage and the pharynx) opening; including tongue exercises. It is important to note that this technique is used only briefly while the patient's swallow reflex returns to original state. The exercises were not to be done when eating or drinking.

I was given another appointment on Wednesday 14 December 2016 at the Adult Speech & Language Therapy to continue with the exercises.

****

Wednesday 14 December 2016 – Rehab Nithbank, Self-referral

FOR SOME UNKNOWN REASON my osteoarthritis became so acute and my balance generally was not good and my ability to walk became slower. I returned to the Rehah Nithbank on a self-referral. My left hip had worsened and my GP referred me to the Orthopaedic Department at the DGRI (the branch of medicine dealing with the correction of deformities of bones or muscles) for consideration of a hip replacement. The Consultant requested my permission to give me a steroid injection into my hip joint. I declined and explained that I was allergic to most medication due to my blood type (Rh negative) as I was not sure what my reaction to the injection would be. He referred me back to my GP who explained that I would benefit from the injection and he would be happy to give it. I consented and it made the world of difference.

I explained to the Rehab Nithbank that I did not think that the hip situation was related to my stroke. Later, my GP also gave me steroid injections in both my knees. These injections alleviated the pain in my hip, knees and legs though my walking was not so good (but I reminded myself, and do remind myself, that I am one year and a few months to 90!)

****

FIVE

Monday 09 January 2017 – Audiology
THE YEAR BEGAN with my attendance at the Hard of Hearing, a service provided for by a charity within the DGRI in Bankend Road. They carried out the usual updating of my existing hearing aids, checking and a supply of spare batteries. After this appointment several other appointments were arranged at the Gilbrae Medical Centre on 13 and 28 March and also 23 May 2017. I continued to use the same hearing aids since the stroke had not caused deterioration of my hearing.

The Gilbrae practice provides, via Dumfries and Galloway Health Board staff, a full range of Health Visiting, Midwifery and District Nursing Services. Community Psychiatric and Community Learning Disability Nursing Services are also available as required. The Surgery is situated in Georgetown.

Audiology is the branch of science and medicine that is concerned with hearing and balance, especially impaired hearing. The evaluation of hearing defects and the rehabilitation of those who have such defects. The next step entailed an audiological evaluation to assess the extent of the hearing loss sustained whether by accident, stroke or other circumstances.

****

Monday 09 January 2017 – Orthotics
I was given an appointment on the above date to finalise the ankle boots. I was seen by Rachel Jenkinson, though Jackie Wright was always present at these appointments, regardless of the member of the Team was taking on the service. On this

occasion I was given an information sheet: "Advice for patients wearing Renace footwear" which also gave instruction on how to look after your footwear.

It was interesting to note that this information covered a number of things, which were unlike what one normally does in caring for shoes: Day to Day Wearing, Cleaning, If your footwear becomes wet, repairs, and Re-ordering.

****

Tuesday 14 February 2017 – Endoscopy
I HAD THE SYMPTOMS OF DYSPHAGIA (a problem with swallowing food).   Although this is classified under "symptoms and signs" in ICD-10, the term is sometimes used as a condition in its own right. A thin area of narrowing in the lower esophagus can intermittently cause difficulty swallowing solid foods.
Despite my assurances to my GP that I was handling the situation well by diet control, liquidising my food (my daughter had also given me an excellent liquidiser/blender), he was not satisfied. He explained that I could choke and such would entail an emergency situation, and he was not comfortable with that.   He made a referral and my appointment was arranged for 03 March 2017 for a one day Admission to Hospital, at the Day Surgery United. This was, in fact, a preventative measure, so I was told. I also received a lot of literature on Speech-language and the pathologist also helped me with speaking and swallowing problems.

The Endoscopy procedure involved a tiny tube inserted down my throat to give a view of the internal parts of my body. There were three Nurses, the Lead player who inserted the tube and two other members of the Team – all with gentle hands as their speech.

The whole process took only ten minutes and when it was over I could not help remarking:

"I do not know what I was worried about. Its not anywhere near like having a baby."

****

Wednesday 22 February 2017 – Rehab Nithbank, Recall discharge

I WAS INVITED ON THE ABOVE DATE and this appointment was more like a review of everything that had taken place before, my progress in Physiotherapy, Occupational Therapy and Nursing on the ongoing issue with dysphasia (language disorder marked by deficiency in the generation of speech), examining my weight (there was no weight loss), and my blood pressure was normal.

Gillian Young, the Lead player in the *finale,* told me that I was discharged from the Rehah Nithbank, and that she would send a letter to my GP explaining my progress.

****

THE IN-BETWEEN ITEM was a letter dated 27 April 2017 advising me on the approach on the waiting list of the day of surgery for my left eye.

****

March 2017 - Keeping Well at Home

I WAS INVITED by Wendy Copeland, Service Manager, in the Nithsdale Locality to join the Nithsdale Public Participation and Engagement Group. The Group was Chaired by Emma McRobert, Project Officer, and after several discussions we reached the consensus that going forward the new model for Nithsdale would be "Nithsdale in Partnership - Keeping Well at Home." The purpose of the Group was to work together to make the communities the best place to live, be active, safe, healthy in fulfilled lives by promoting independence, choice and control.

I attended the first meeting on Tuesday 11 April 2017, followed by other meetings. A number of points were discussed including using a range of existing structures. The Group sought to co-ordinate a variety of methods to actively engage and promote participation from people of all ages and abilities and to reach those who would not normally come forward to share their views and ideas. There was also a discussion around linking in with more national information. Since then the group has been disbanded however, having further discussions with Wendy and Emma, I am looking forward to being involved in future work developing the Community Rehabilitation model, by sitting on a short life working group that will be formed later in 2018.

These two invitations, from Wendy Copeland as that extended by Chris Wallace, were very important to me because they made me feel that I was not 'redundant' or relegated to the 'useless' heap. For some, not being regarded as redundant is good for the morale, despite the after effects of having had a stroke, not to mention my advanced age.

****

OUT OF THE BLUE   one April morning I got a telephone call from Ann-Marie Budyn inviting me to meet Father Nazarius Mgungwe, a Roman Catholic Priest from Malawi who lived in Oxford, England. Anna called at my home, collected me and drove us to Lock Arthur Farm Shop [Note 10.] Father Nazarius Mgungwe seemed rather familiar to me but I could not place him – I have indicated above that since my stroke my memory had become rather weak. Gradually my memory of the Father began to open up. Then I asked him:

"Did you baptise a baby called Miquel Van Rooyen?" He replied that he had in Stoke-on-Trent. Then it all rushed back to me. Miquel was my eldest brother's (deceased) great grand son. The baptism took place at St George and St Martins Church in 2008. It was a happy occasion when a good number of members of the family had gathered together.

Sadly, in 2009, members of the family gathered again at the Hope Hospital in Manchester, England, when Roxanne, grandmother of Miquel and youngest daughter of my eldest brother was admitted at Hope Hospital for a brain haemorrhage. The life support machine was switched off and Roxanne passed on at the tender age of 48. Father Nazarius also conducted the funeral service of Roxanne at the Crematorium in Macclesfield. My memory of that occasion: Father Nazarius had placed the Cross and the Holy Bible on Roxanne's casket which I found rather comforting.

Anna's out of the blue telephone invitation was truly 'awesome'.

****

Tuesday 23 May 2017 – Colonoscopy

MY COLONOSCOPY APPOINTMENT was booked for 27 April, it was performed by a lady doctor and lasted approximately 30 minutes. Medication was given into my vein to make me feel relaxed and drowsy. I was asked to lie on my left side on the examining table. During the colonoscopy the doctor used a colonoscope, a long flexible, tubular, instrument about ½-inch in diameter that transmitted an image of the

Note 10: A working Community in the South West of Scotland, which includes men and women with learning disabilities; and where children are guided towards greater independence through development of self-help skills.

lining of the colon so the doctor could examine it for abnormalities. A colonoscope is inserted through the rectum and advanced to the other end of the sigmoid colon (large intestine). I watched the whole process on a screen. The colonoscopy revealed that there was no problem.

The appointment letter included an explanation "Preparing for Colonoscopy". Perhaps the only uncomfortable part of the procedure was the bowel preparation before the surgery as it had to be emptied prior to the surgery by drinking Movieprep solution contained in sachets and mixed with lukewarm water. This also involved minimal fasting.

****

Wednesday 24 May 2017 – Eye Test
I made an appointment to visit SpecSavers as advised by the Ophthalmology Department. On this pre-surgery appointment they were most helpful, particularly the *Fundi* who gave me the eye test. Despite that they were an organisation separate from the DGRI Hospital, the spirit of 'Liaison', or 'unity' if you like, was apparent.

****

Wednesday 24 May 2017 – Ophthalmology
I RECEIVED ANOTHER APPOINTMENT to attend at the Ophthalmology Department for a further eye test. This was carried out by one of the Ophthalmologists: shining a light into the eye and measuring the refractive error by evaluating the movement of the light reflected by my retina back

through my pupil. To examine my visual acuity, I was given numbing drops in my eyes and the doctor measured my eye pressure; checked the health of my eyes by using several lights to evaluate the front of the eye and inside of each eye. My eyes were also dilated with eye drops; evaluated the muscles that control eye movement by watching my eye movements as my eyes followed a moving object, pen/small light. He also looked for muscle weakness, poor control or coordination. I was asked to identify different letters of the alphabet printed on a chart (Snellen Chart, named after the Dutch ophthalmologist Herman Snellen who developed the chart in 1862). The examination determined that I needed surgery, particularly in my left eye.

Another appointment was arranged for 08 June 2017 following a similar procedure, by a different doctor, one of the Team. And, it was determined that I was to have cataract surgery to both eyes. This was followed by a letter on 23 June, 2017, letting me know that I was
getting closer to the date on the waiting list for the surgery procedure. Finally an appointment was set for 29 June 2017 when various tests for cataract surgery assessment were carried out.

****

Friday 09 June 2017 - Dermatology
I RECEIVED AN APPOINTMENT to attend the hospital where I was seen by the Registrar at the Outpatients. This was occasioned by my request to my GP for Psoriasis that had bothered me for a good number of years. The Registrar was more concerned about a black mole on my right groin that had grown bigger and bigger over the years to the size of a two-penny piece.

Thursday 13 June 2017 – Stroke Rehabilitation, Falls Prevention Programme Classes

SINCE I HAD MENTIONED TO MY GP my lack of balance, I received a letter from the Senior Physiotherapist, letting me know that I was to attend, on the above date, Falls Prevention Programme Classes commencing on the above date from 1:00 pm to 2:30 pm. The classes were held at the Cluden Cardiac Unit, Cluden East, Crichton Hall, where I had first met Lynn Robertson though she was not part of this team.

The exercises consisted of the ones the Nurse had showed me when she called on me and others I had never done before. There were others done while seated with yellow rubber bands and we wore plain white goggles (apparently for protection to the eyes, since someone had got hurt before). As I have said, they looked after every aspect of my body!

I attended the classes for six weeks and this was followed by an appointment to attend at Rehab Nithbank on 19 June 2017 where the Lead Physiotherapist completed an assessment test for a final time. She gave me very good ratings and I was discharged, after participating and enjoying the usual 'social club' atmosphere.

****

Tuesday 13 June 2017 – Loss of Balance
FOR SOME UNKNOWN REASON I found my legs giving way and found it increasingly difficult to walk. This also affected my balance. I went to see my GP and he suggested a 'walker', also known as a 'rollator'. I was soon visited by a Nurse who brought along with her a rollator on loan to me for 4 weeks with instructions on how to use it. She also showed me some

exercises I was to do, designed to counteract the lack of balance. I faithfully carried out the exercises and also took the rollator and walked to the beautiful Dock Park by the River Nith. On my first walk, I managed to walk for three quarters of an hour including the return walk. This was later increased to one and one-half hours both ways comfortably.

I should point out that a good number of women on my grandmother' side (my mother's mother) of the family had suffered from weakness in their legs and a few of them when they reached age 65-70 could not
walk at all. Particularly in the village where wheelchairs were unknown they had to be carried around. Whenever I feel the weakness in my legs I try to remind myself that it could be genetic, but this is a situation I am not prepared to accept.

****

Monday 19 June 2017 - Rehab Gym Assessment
I RECEIVED A LETTER from Lead player telling me that an appointment had been booked on the above date to complete the assessment tests for the final time. The letter also explained that in
looking at information on the longer term benefits of the exercise programme the assessment was important. The assessment was carried out but I was asked to call again on 05 September 2017, when on this latter date I was discharged.

****

Thursday 29 June 2017 - Assessment
I received a letter dated 23 June 2017 telling me that the date on the waiting list was imminent for a procedure to be carried out for my left eye and on the above date various tests for cataract surgery assessment were carried out. This was

followed by a letter telling me that an appointment for admission to Hospital – Day Care (Ward 17) was
arranged for Tuesday 04 July 2017 at 8:15. Along with this
was an information sheet on the usual things on pre "Do and
Don't".

On the appointed date I met the Leading *Fundi* who was to
carry out the surgery. The gentlest of hands prepared me for
the surgery before the *Fundi* was to commence his skill; and
a nurse sat next to me holding my hands under a covering and
told me that I should squeeze her hand should I feel any pain.
Another nurse was on my right, and I believe the *Fundi* was
behind my head. I thought I was still waiting for the surgery
to be carried out; for I felt no pain or discomfort whatsoever.
Then it was over.

This was followed by a letter telling me that I was to attend
the hospital the following day (Wednesday 05 July). On this
day a "reading test" on the Snellen Chart was carried out on
my left eye by another *Fundi* member of the Team (post
operative refraction). It was not a matter of:
 "I see", said the blind man (as he hit a lamp post!) but it was
like a "window opened to the world". I could read the Snellen
Chart. A miracle had been performed!

I arranged an appointment for 27 July 2017 with SpecSavers
for glasses as advised by the Ophthalmology Department. My
eyes were tested and I was given a pair of glasses but my sight
was not 'balanced' pending surgery to the right eye.

****

**Tuesday 04 July 2017 at 8:15 - Post operative refraction
record**
I received the usual appointment letter telling me that an

Admission to Hospital – Day Care (Ward 17) was arranged for the above date. Along with this was an information sheet on the usual things on pre "Do and Don't".

Then I met the Leading *Fundi* who was to carry out the surgery. The gentlest of hands prepared me for the surgery before the *Fundi* was to commence his skill; and a nurse sat next to me holding my hands under a covering and told me that I should squeeze her hand should I feel any pain. Another nurse was on my right, and I believe the *Fundi* was behind my head. I thought I was still waiting for the surgery to be carried out; for I felt no pain or discomfort whatsoever. Then it was over.

This was followed by a letter telling me that I was to attend the hospital the following day (Wednesday 05 July). On this day a "reading test" on the Snellen Chart was carried out on my left eye by another *Fundi* member of the Team. It was not a matter of: "I see", said the blind man (as he hit a lamp post!) but it was like a "window opened to the world". I could read the Snellen Chart. A miracle had been performed!

I arranged an appointment for 27 July 2017 with SpecSavers for glasses as advised by the Ophthalmology Department. My eyes were tested and I was given a pair of glasses but my sight was not 'balanced' pending surgery to the right eye.

****

Tuesday 18 July 2017 – Excision Biopsy

I have indicated above that the Registrar was more concerned about the "two-penny" size mole on my right groin. At a later date I received an Outpatient Appointment to attend at the Dermatology Department for an Excision biopsy on the right hip. The surgery was carried out by a Sister and it involved 7 stitches which were removed after 10 days by a Practice Nurse at my medical 'home base'. The surgery was painless and took no more than 20 minutes.

This was followed by a letter dated 25 July, 2017 from the Consultant Dermatologist advising me that the lesion removed from my right groin area was a "seborrhoeic keratosis", it was a common harmless skin growth, and that no further treatment was required.

****

OUT OF THE BLUE I had a phone call from Liane Henderson asking me if I would be willing to pose as a 'pretend patient' in a little drama. I was rather intrigued since I have always loved drama and 'theatricals' ever since I was a child. Katrina Logie (Kasia) and Tina McNaught came on the first occasion when they explained that they were setting up a new Service and the purpose was "To document in assessing how long a first visit to a patient would take to complete." On the second occasion I was visited by Carolina Mroczkowski and Liane Henderson when they completed the assessment.

I very much enjoyed the company of these NHS ladies (as I always do). They are so inspiring and full of laughter - what is life without a laugh?

****

Tuesday 08 August 2017 - Ophthalmology
MY APPOINTMENT for Admission to Hospital – Day Care (Ward 17) was arranged for the above date for surgery to my right eye and that the same *Fundi* would carry out the surgery. Along with this was an information sheet on the usual things on pre "Do and Don't". A letter was sent to my GP

saying that there would be no further follow-up to this surgery.

The Nurse who looked after things in the waiting room asked where I lived and whether I lived alone. I told her and confirmed that I lived alone. She offered me a sandwich to take home - how considerate! She even offered me a choice of cheese/tomato, ham or egg. This was done while I was waiting for the taxi to take me home. [During most of the eye services involved my daughter picking me up or ordering a taxi.]

****

WHILE THE ABOVE WAS GOING ON at Nithsdale Mills where I lived there were other activities organised by Loreburn Housing. They had appointed Hollie Mitchell. On Friday 23 June 2017 was the first, a visit to the Bowling Green. There were 15 of us collected by two enthusiastic and helpful drivers of Premier Taxis (Dumfries). The vans were equipped to take the physically challenged, some with their rollators.

We were not in any way coerced to take part in the game, yet somehow found ourselves participating in the mood of the event, despite the slightly inclement weather. There was shelter and the hospitality of tea, coffee and biscuits.

This lovely, charming young woman provided excellent service. She was dependable, unassuming but caring and compassionate and she carried out the responsibility of looking after 15 "ol' dears" without any trouble at all. This event was, at a later date, followed by a visit to Threave Gardens (a reminder of the Edinburgh Botanical Gardens and Kew Gardens, London). There were also other visits to theatres, cinema and various other outings.

SIX

Thursday 02 November 2017 – Health Well-being Team
HAVING COMPLETED ALL I needed to do at the Rehab Gym and had been assessed by the Lead player, the latter arranged an appointment for Lindsay Murdoch, Community Link Worker, Healthy Connections, Nithsdale Health and Well-being Team of the NHS (DG Health and Social Care) to carry out, what I would call 'ongoing care'. She called on me on the above date and brought along with her a bundle of literature covering numerous subjects on: Activities & Initiatives; Dumfries Get Together; Dumfries & Galloway Over 50's Group; Dumfries Day Centre; Dumfries Walking Club; Dance and Fitness – Studio 3, with 12 fitness items to choose from; Easy Chair Based Exercises; and See Hear Project. As I have indicated in previous chapters, they covered everything from head to toe, and once you are in the 'safety net' they do everything possible to see that you remain within the 'safety net' – what I would call "service beyond the call of duty".

The Dumfries & Galloway Health Well-being Team carries the logo of a tree with many flowering branches made up of "all hands on" – whoever designed the logo certainly carried a holistic vision on the care NHS gives in the aspect of health and well-being.

Lindsay also arranged for the replacement of my broken Clip-on Raised Toilet Seat.

****

Friday 17 November 2017
On this day Lindsay made a follow up visit and brought with her a 12-page listing of social events; she also brought a 7-

page listing on matters of reading and discussion groups; language; poetry; history; travel and holiday. On the afternoon of this day the toilet seat was delivered - what service!

I mentioned to her that I was interested in Tea Dancing (despite the weakness of my legs!). She gave me information on two places, Hole in the Wall in the High Street, Dumfries; and the Dance Group at the Summerhill Community Centre. On the weakness of my legs, my reasoning is that: If Pistorius (without legs) could run a marathon and become a champion, so too, I can dance without legs!

I made several telephone calls to see what I could select for my "regular recreation", visited some of the areas where the events were taking place, and to see how far away they were located from my place of residence.

I can now no longer sit behind the wheel and drive for miles – like I used to say to my friends:
    "I am driving to the end of the world." And, they would ask:
    "Where is the end of the world?" I replied:
    "I shall send you a postcard when I get there."
I once drove from London to Inverness – the farthest I can go is 15 miles but I constantly remind myself that I am one year and four months to 90 and during the 70 years of my impeccable driving licence I had driven thousands of miles – everything passes away...

I chose some activity for each day of the week from the following list:
On the social aspect -
Dumfries Get Together and Over 50s Group, involving concerts, plays and other social activities;

On the Body fitness:
Yoga, Tai Chi, Chair Based Exercises, and Tea Dance; and in addition to the above I faithfully do the exercises which I was taught at the Rehab Gym plus what I have done over the years.

****

Monday 27 November 2017- Visibility
I WAS VISITED AT HOME by Mia Glendinning. This was as a result of Lindsay Murdoch's follow-up on my eyesight and hearing. I had made the point that my hearing aids had been prescribed for tinnitus that had bothered me for a long time. Therefore, the hearing aids were for a mild hearing problem and they needed to be stronger since my hearing had become weaker.

Aside from being helpful on the follow-up on my hearing aids and eyesight, we had much to talk about as Mia was bubbly and interesting. She was from Johannesburg, South Africa, the place where Francis Argente, father of Lorna, my daughter, died at the tender age of 38 on a Harley Davidson in a motor accident in 1967 (see *Blantyre and Yawo Women*, chapter 13).

Friday 08 December 2017 – Cresswell Redevelopment Project
THIS WAS A DAY OF "history-in-the-making" when certain services at the DGRI, Nithbank Road, were moved to the new DGRI hospital at Cardenbridge. No doubt they were well-organised in advance of the event but I could not help thinking about the moving of patients in different categories. One of the departments to move was the Maternity wing and I thought about possibly some babies in incubators being moved among the categories.

Also connected to this move was the Cresswell Redevelopment Project (CRP). The plan was that the present Maternity wing of the DGRI at Nithbank Road was to be turned into premises to accommodate several departments of NHS including the Rehabilitation Unit at Nithbank.

Two persons had been invited, Elaine Smith, who had also attended the Rehabilitation Unit at Nithbank, and myself to serve as Patient Representatives on the CRP. The invitation was extended by Chris Wallace, Day Services Manager - Community Rehabilitation/ Bladder, Bowel and Pelvic Floor Health (BBH)/ Building Healthy Communities, Nithsdale Locality, Community Health and Social Care, for his department.

This involved attendance of meetings at the Crichton Conference Hall, with ideas for the new premises. According to the discussions at the meetings of the CRP, plans presented, and points raised, the one shortcoming of the Rehabilitation Unit at Nithbank would be addressed and rectified, that is: The premises at Nithbank were not designed for the purpose or service provided, that of 'Rehabilitation'. Despite this shortcoming, efforts were made to make the premises suitable for the purpose. As far as the service provided to patients was concerned, I would comment, and this is seconded to by my colleague, Elaine Smith, that *it was second to none* (see comments in the Epilogue below).

Notably, while Elaine and I faithfully attended the meetings at the Crichton Conference Hall, there were no attendances by any others to represent patients in other departments of NHS.

****

WE HAD OUR LAST MEETING on 16 May 2018. The purpose of the meeting was to inform the Nithbank Team on what Elaine and I had gained from the Cresswell Meetings and our experience on consultation.

My part was to commence by commending the service I received at the Rehabilitation Unit, Nithbank (Rehab Nithbank) from all the personnel I came into contact with in the various things that were done to repair my *broken temple.* Elaine shared my opinion of Rehab Nithbank that: *the service was second to none.*

In welcoming the proposals of the Cresswell Project to improve the new premises, there was a shortcoming that I found: the premises of the Rehab Nithbank where these excellent services were performed, had not been purposely designed or built for rehabilitation and some of the facilities were not offering their maximum results. Again, credit goes to the personnel who did so much to make the premises workable.

I then passed on to Elaine to outline the criticisms of Nithbank premises:

She commenced by saying that at the first meeting it was explained to everyone that the purpose of the workshop was to evaluate the existing designs, and a key aspect of this evaluation was the functionality of the building. That the several negative issues she had raised regarding the rehab unit at Nithbank, was not about critiquing the service, as the service she had received had been outstanding. That because the building hadn't been purposely designed for a rehabilitation unit, it resulted in some facilities not being able to offer their maximum potential. She then went on to explain the nature of the shortcomings

On the suggestions for the Draft Design:
After that first meeting we had received an email from Karen who worked on the design team, she asked for staff and patients to provide
examples in pictures of good and/or bad designs of certain areas within the building. Elaine replied by submitting several images suggestive of what the future plan should consist of.

There was a change of the Original plans. Chris had received a draft of the plans, when he showed them to Rose and myself we were all disappointed. As the waiting area had been placed in the corridor. So

Chris set up a meeting with the architects and design team, he put forward our concerns with regards the location of the waiting area. As a result, new plans were drafted and thankfully our concerns were addressed, and the waiting area was moved in to a more private location with natural light as well! Another example of our wee voices being listened to!

The Outcome:
As patients Elaine and I were more than happy with the outcome of the final draft Design Statement. However, I was also concerned about facilities for the staff such as parking area, etc., things we take for granted. The staff should be considered no less because they look after people.

Like any other organisation, the NHS is just a shell. It is the people who work in NHS in the different departments that make NHS what it is: an organisation that looks after people when they are at their lowest ebb. Employees of any organisation are 'partners'. Without them there is nothing. We live in a system that tend to give more credence to those who provide the infrastructure.

I mentioned that I was deeply honoured that I had been invited to represent patients at the Cresswell Meetings. It made me feel that in spite of my condition (not to mention my age!) I was considered not redundant but still useful.

Rehabilitation means healing without medication. Not everybody can take medication.   I personally have great difficulty in taking medication because my blood is a rare type Rh D Negative. Some medication has proved to have a horrendous effect on me. I also have had to monitor my diet over the years and make constant changes in what I eat, otherwise my body rejects certain types of food within 10 minutes of eating.

Elaine summarised her Experience:
AT THE TIME CHRIS ASKED ME to be a patient representative on this project, I had just had an occupational health assessment and was told at that assessment that I would not be fit to return to work. My job made up such a huge part of my identity, returning to work had been
one of the main goals that I had set at rehab – that and walking my dog Dexter again! As a result, I was left feeling deflated, that I had nothing to offer society and I was lost with regards a goal to work towards. So Chris' request was a huge boost to my confidence and it helped make me feel I still had something to offer. Throughout the project, I felt listened to and was made to feel that what I had to say was informative and helpful. As I said before, this was validated when I saw several of the issues I had raised about the Nithbank building had been taken on board and the new designs reflected the necessary changes for improvement. This was especially the

case at this last meeting, my previous comments on the outdoor space had well and truly been taken on board. When the architect unveiled the outdoor space, I can honestly say I got a lump in my throat and it brought tears to my eyes. He had designed it so that there were several different terrains and gradients and it was in an enclosed safe environment. But there was also a secondary outdoor space nearer to the road, which, once the enclosed space had been mastered, would be the next phase of outdoor therapy! It is exactly what I had envisioned and would have wanted for my own therapy, so to see it designed for the new premises.

Where future patients would benefit from it was amazing! So overall it has been a positive and uplifting experience which I am grateful to have been a part of. It was a privilege to represent past and future patients, and an honour to be able to contribute to an improved rehabilitation unit for future staff and patients.

****

I HAD SUGGESTED to Elaine that we met at the new DGRI Hospital so that she could have the opportunity of visiting the place. I had already visited twice. Sadly, Elaine was in great pain and she had to go home after our discussion. That she came to meet me when she was in such pain, was highly commendable. I would like to mention that Elaine has been very helpful to me, she is highly intelligent and able to grasp the intrinsic aspect of any subject. She made a great contribution to the Cresswell Project.

At the new DGRI I was welcomed at the Reception desk where the Receptionist was most helpful and she found an empty ward (waiting for a patient to come in). She said she was taking me on a shorter walk but for me it was a very long walk - the hospital is massive.

It is comprised of all single rooms and patients do not have to share; very well designed with all facilities for taking blood pressure, etc. and the walls are of a very pale turquoise: A truly *5 star plus* mini bedsit, with toilet en suite.

****

I CONTINUED TO ATTEND the Bahá'í meetings alternating the venue at different households as hosted by different Bahá'í members. I further learned that since the inception of the Bahá'í Faith in the Nineteenth Century, a growing number of people have found in the teachings of Bahá'u'lláh a compelling vision of a better world. Many have drawn insights from these teachings—for example, on the oneness of humanity, and on the equality of women and men, on the elimination of prejudice, on the harmony of science and religion—and have sought to apply Bahá'í principles to their lives and work. Others have gone further and have decided to join the Bahá'í community and participate in its efforts to contribute directly to the realisation of Bahá'u'lláh's stupendous vision for humanity's coming of age.

At the Bahá'í meetings I met many interesting persons. There were also visiting speakers who came from other parts of the world, aside from other local residents of Dumfries who much brightened my life and inspired me in more ways than one. Among the people I met at the Bahá'í meetings was Moshira El Azzawi Maddison from whom I got the impression that we had met in another life, possibly in the days of the Pharaohs. Perhaps to some this may sound a little far-fetched but I strongly believe that each one of us, including you and I, at some point in history, came from the same parents. Our ancestors live on in us and in the same way we shall live on in posterity. I have never doubted that this could be proved by DNA.

Based on this belief I ordered my DNA through Ancestry. I could not wait to see who I was related to and what historical context would be revealed over the centuries. Since my genetic make-up is from three sources: African (Malawi), Northern European (France), and Asian (India), I was looking towards these areas but I was shocked to find that I am related to people (4th to 6th cousins) in Africa: North, Ivory Coast/Ghana, Nigeria, Benin/Togo; Europe: West, South, East,

Scandinavia, Iberia Peninsula, European Jewish, Great Britain: Scotland, Wales, Ireland, Northwest Russia, Caucasus; and Asia: South, Central,
East Polynesia; and hundreds others which would take months to go through. Suffice to say the 'human race is one' and the difference in skin colour or cultures really does not tell us much about what we really are (see *Difference*).

****

THROUGH VENUS CAREW I attended the screening of the film *Mercy's Blessing* at The Stove, Dumfries, Scotland, on Friday 15th June. The film was made in Malawi by May Taherzadeh. I was born and raised in Malawi and the film greatly moved me. In the 30 minutes of the film it captures the message of social injustice, the importance of education, gender equality and education, and the power of choice.

The story reflect the 'sadness' of the situation on education in that part of the world, especially for girls. The girl child does not have a choice. The choice may come when she passes girlhood and by her own efforts she can strive to achieve what she wants. The power of choice is one that can come from adults and institutions to keep the girl child in school.

May Taherzadeh went to Malawi as a baby with her parents in 1976 and lived there until 1996. She now lives in the Netherlands with her Dutch husband and their four children, one boy and three girls. One of the girls was adopted as an infant from a Malawi orphanage and now she is 6 years old.

Addendum:
The most common IS include: Transient Ischemic attack (TIA); Thrombotic stroke (TS); Embotic stroke (ES); Intracerebral Haemorrhage (IH); Subarachnoid Haemorrhage (SH).

TIA— also known as a mini stroke — is a brief period of symptoms similar to those you'd have in a stroke, a temporary decrease in blood supply to part of one's brain causes TIAs, which often last less than five minutes. A TIA doesn't leave lasting symptoms because the blockage is temporary. Seek emergency care even if your symptoms seem to clear up. Having a TIA puts you at greater risk of having a full-blown stroke, causing permanent damage later. If you've had a TIA, it means there's likely a partially blocked or narrowed artery leading to your brain or a clot source in the heart.

TS – A blood clot (thrombus) forms in one of the arteries that supply blood to the brain. Like an ischemic stroke, a clot may be caused by fatty deposits (plaque) that build up in arteries and cause reduced blood flow (atherosclerosis) or other artery conditions.

It is not possible to tell if one is having a stroke or a TIA based only on your symptoms. Up to half of people whose symptoms appear to go away actually have had a stroke causing brain damage.

ES – occurs when a blood clot or other debris forms away from your brain – commonly in one's heart – and is swept through the bloodstream to lodge in narrower brain arteries. This type of blood clot is called an embolus.

IH - In an intracerebral haemorrhage, a blood vessel in the brain bursts and spills into the surrounding brain tissue, damaging brain cells. Brain cells beyond the leak are deprived of blood and also damaged. High
blood pressure, trauma, vascular malformations, use of blood-thinning medications and other conditions may cause an intracerebral haemorrhage.

SH - In a subarachnoid haemorrhage, an artery on or near the surface of your brain bursts and spills into the space between the surface of your brain and your skull. This bleeding is often signaled by a sudden, severe headache. A subarachnoid haemorrhage is commonly caused by the bursting of a small sack-shaped or berry-shaped outpouching on an
artery known as an aneurysm. After the haemorrhage, the blood vessels in your brain may widen and narrow erratically (vasospasm), causing brain cell damage by further limiting blood flow.

Generally people who have had a stroke experience changes in behaviour and self-care ability in varying degrees, they may need help with grooming and daily chores; some may become withdrawn and less social while others become more impulsive. TIA, also known as a mini stroke — is a brief period of symptoms similar to those you'd have in a stroke, a temporary decrease in blood supply to part of one's brain causes TIAs, which often last less than five minutes. A TIA doesn't leave lasting symptoms because the blockage is temporary. Seek emergency care even if your symptoms seem to clear up. Having a TIA puts you at greater risk of having a full-blown stroke, causing permanent damage later. If you've had a TIA, it means there's likely a partially blocked or narrowed artery leading to your brain or a clot source in the heart.

TS – A blood clot (thrombus) forms in one of the arteries that supply blood to the brain. Like an ischemic stroke, a clot may be caused by fatty deposits (plaque) that build up in arteries and cause reduced blood flow (atherosclerosis) or other artery conditions.

It's not possible to tell if one is having a stroke or a TIA based only on your symptoms. Up to half of people whose symptoms appear to go away actually have had a stroke causing brain damage.

ES – occurs when a blood clot or other debris forms away from your brain – commonly in one's heart – and is swept through the bloodstream to lodge in narrower brain arteries. This type of blood clot is called an embolus.

IH - In an intracerebral haemorrhage, a blood vessel in the brain bursts and spills into the surrounding brain tissue, damaging brain cells. Brain cells beyond the leak are deprived of blood and also damaged. High blood pressure, trauma, vascular malformations, use of blood-thinning medications and other conditions may cause an intracerebral haemorrhage.

SH - In a subarachnoid haemorrhage, an artery on or near the surface of your brain bursts and spills into the space

between the surface of your brain and your skull.   This bleeding is often signaled by a sudden,
severe headache. A subarachnoid haemorrhage is commonly caused by the bursting of a small sack-shaped or berry-shaped outpouching on an artery known as an aneurysm. After the haemorrhage, the blood vessels in your brain may widen and narrow erratically (vasospasm), causing brain cell damage by further limiting blood flow.

Generally people who have had strokes experience changes in behaviour and self-care ability in varying degrees, they may need help with grooming and daily chores; some may become withdrawn and less sociable while others become more impulsive.

Epilogue

I believe it is appropriate for me to entitle this book *Broken Temple* following the vision of Moses on Mount Sinai. The main source for the description of the construction of the Tabernacle is in the Old Testament (Exodus 25:31 and 35:40). From the time of the Exodus from Egypt through the conquering of the land of Canaan, the Tabernacle was the portable earthly dwelling place of God amongst the Israelite according to their faith. Symbolic to the body of Jesus was the veil that separated the "Holy Place" and "Holy of Hollies" in the inner shrine which housed the Ark of Covenant: the dwelling place of God. The Tabernacle was also symbolic to the human body as a temple housing the soul on its temporal sojourn. Some 300 years later Solomon's Temple in Jerusalem superseded the Tabernacle as the dwelling place of God (see *The Veil* and *The Promised Land – Companion to The Veil*).

According to my experience, the reality is that having had a stroke you are no longer the person you were before the stroke, mentally and physically, and you see the world in a different light: because the *Temple* broke. If you've had a stroke, your brain will need to relearn some old skills. You'll need a refresher course on things you used to take for granted, like speaking, organising your thoughts, and taking a walk. Perhaps above all, is the feeling that you never lived your life as you ought to have done but wasted it on trivial matters, particularly in caring for those in dire circumstances. The significance of a line from Robert Browning's poem becomes more apparent: *I shall not pass this way again...*

Stroke Rehabilitation (Stroke Rehab) is not only an important part of recovery after a stroke but also indispensable. The goal of a Stroke Rehab programme is to help one relearn lost skills when stroke affected part of the brain, but more so, I found, was to *learn new skills* to enable you to cope with daily life. Rehabilitation gives one 'confidence', enables one to tackle things and regain independence. More so to some, independence is very important.

Occupational therapists will help you practice daily tasks like eating, bathing, and writing. Your physical therapist and other team members will guide you in exercises that strengthen your muscles, improve your coordination, and help you walk - on your own or with a wheelchair or walker (also known as rollator). Physical therapists will work with you on exercises to improve movement, balance, and coordination. Occupational therapists will help you practise daily tasks like eating, bathing, and writing. Speech-language pathologists will help you with speaking and swallowing problems.

Stroke Rehab can help you regain your confidence, independence and improve your quality of life and let you enjoy the things you love. A stroke Rehab program can help your brain to get the job done. It may not reverse the effects of your stroke. But then, in life most things are not reversible. However, your grey matter has an amazing ability to repair and rewire itself. And, what I have called 'ongoing care', aside from the medical aspect, is very important for those in the Octogenarian category.

On the question of 'memory' I found that my memory had been considerably affected by my stroke, particularly on languages. The languages I learned as a toddler, Yawo (my grandmother's language) and ChiChewa, one of the official languages of Malawi (the other is English) have not been affected by the stroke. The languages I learned in later life, Swahili, Portuguese, and French, were almost entirely lost after the stroke.

I learned Swahili in my early teens (through the wife of my uncle who brought her to Malawi from Tanzania). My knowledge of Swahili was also strengthened by my husband, Francis Argente, who came from Dar es Salaam, Tanzania.

Portuguese came naturally, also in my early teens by virtue of our neighbouring country Mozambique (then Portuguese East Africa). I formally learned French when I was 45 at the French Embassy, Cultural Centre, Blantyre, Malawi, where classes were held. My knowledge was confined to written French rather than spoken as I never visited France or pursued the speech aspect though I mastered the language to translate a document from French to English and vice versa.

I also found that the English language (which I began to speak from age 5) had become terribly weak and I forget a word in the middle of a sentence. Also, my daughter has taken me to certain places around Dumfries and some of them I do not remember that I visited them before.

To support this I mention an incident about a friend from Malawi (who now lives in Glastonbury, Somerset). She suffered a stroke just as she was about to have heart surgery. A mutual friend visited her and said that people could not understand what she was saying: she was speaking in *Sena*, an African vernacular language. I understood this because I recalled that *Sena* was the first language she spoke as a toddler.

Strange as it may seem, memories of the distant past remain fast in the mind, more so than of more recent incidents. Perhaps above all is the constant memories of those who have passed on - the longer one lives the more people pass away and leaves one bereft despite that one may be surrounded by 'kindness'. The best way to combat this 'sad aspect of remembering' is to engage in *activity* and meet as many people as possible. And, the "Safety Net" of the NHS with its varied health connections does ensure that there are many activities to choose from.

In my twilight years my 'Broken Temple' followed my 'Broken Heart' in my youth by the loss of my infants but I have been very fortunate in my only surviving child Lorna who gave me reason to go on. She has been daughter, sister, friend, and mother, making up for the missing total of four, hence my spirit is 'unbroken.' I have much to thank God for, through Yeshua, my Mentor and Saviour for placing so much 'kindness' around me.

Broken Temple is a tribute to the United Kingdom National Health Service (NHS) and personnel...in particular a highly sympathetic account of the Community Rehabilitation, Nithbank, Dumfries & Galloway Royal Infirmary (DGRI) of the NHS...highlights its care and active management entailing the treatment of disabling conditions and prevention of secondary disorders...a personal account of the author's experience with having a stroke...

www.ingramcontent.com/pod-product-compliance
Lightning Source LLC
Chambersburg PA
CBHW071120210326
41519CB00020B/6357